MANAGED CARE:
INTEGRATING THE DELIVERY AND FINANCING OF HEALTH CARE

PART C

D1712063

STUDY MANUAL

The Health Insurance Association of America
Washington, D.C. 20004-1109

© 1998 by the Health Insurance Association of America
All rights reserved. Published 1998
Printed in the United States of America

ISBN 1-879143-47-x

TABLE OF CONTENTS

TO THE STUDENT

Our textbook *Managed Care: Integrating the Delivery and Financing of Health Care, Part C* will further your knowledge of the basic concepts of managed care, building on Parts A and B.

The *Managed Care, Part C* textbook has been written by industry contributors who are specialists in their fields. This study manual has been developed by HIAA Insurance Education staff—persons skilled and experienced in the field of adult and industry education.

We hope that your participation in the HIAA Education Program will contribute to the broadening of your capabilities and the advancement of your career.

HOW TO USE THIS STUDY MANUAL

There are two types of knowledge you need to successfully pass this course: knowledge of the subject and knowledge of testing techniques. This study manual is designed to help you succeed in both.

However, please keep in mind that the Study Manual is not a substitute for the textbook. Remember that you are supplying the answers yourself—and that you could be wrong or be interpreting the question a different way from someone else! It would be best to compare answers with another student if possible. The Study Manual is a summary of the textbook and asks the types of questions likely to appear on the examination. But the exam may want more detail, or possibly ask something that was not covered in the Study Manual. Nothing can replace a detailed knowledge of the textbook itself.

SUGGESTIONS FOR STUDY— KNOWLEDGE OF THE SUBJECT

Examine the textbook and study manual thoroughly and set up a schedule for completing all material at least a week before the scheduled examination. You may need to divide longer chapters into smaller study units.

Time:

We suggest you set aside one week for every 20 pages. The time you need for each chapter will vary depending on your previous knowledge of the subject. However, we cannot caution you enough on one point: HIAA textbooks try to give a picture of *industry* practice as a whole— your own company may do things differently from the description in the textbook.

Steps in Studying:

1) Read the Key Terms. Which ones don't you know? Are you clear on the differences between similar terms?

2) Read the chapter completely but quickly.

3) Re-read the Key Terms. Are there still any you are not sure of? If so, look them up in the chapter or the glossary. Can you define the differences between similar terms? If not, look them up in the chapter or glossary.

4) Answer the questions in this Study Manual without using the textbook.

5) Re-read the chapter again, more thoroughly, checking your answers in the Study Manual as you go. Fill in answers to questions you could not answer before and change answers to questions you got wrong before. (Questions in the Study Manual are in approximately the same order as the subjects appear in the textbook.) It would be helpful if you used a different color pen to correct the Study Manual (red instead of black, for instance). Then, when you use the Study Manual to study for the examination, you will know exactly where your weaknesses are and what to spend your time studying.

6) As you re-read the chapter thoroughly and check your Study Manual answers, make a note of terms or concepts that are still not clear, even after checking the textbook. Are there any parts of the textbook you think are ambiguous? Compare notes with others in your company taking the same course, your education representative, or someone who is an expert in that area in your company.

7) As you re-read the chapter thoroughly, can you find material in the textbook that has not been covered in the Study Manual? Make a note of it.

8) A week before the examination, re-read the Study Manual. Check your knowledge of the Key Terms. Look at the notes you made of material that was not covered by the Study Manual. Ask yourself what questions you might expect to find on the examination.

Stick to your schedule of 20 pages a week. Do not leave reading or studying until the last minute.

What Should You Study?

The number of questions on the examination are distributed using two criteria: the length of the treatment in the text and the importance of the subject. It may take five pages to describe a complicated concept, but only one page to describe an equally important, but not as complicated, subject. If we distributed questions on the basis of length alone, the concept that took five pages would have five times as many questions. If we distributed questions on the basis of importance alone, each subject would have an equal number of questions. We distribute questions based on both criteria: length and importance. So the concept that took five pages to explain might have slightly more questions than the equally important subject that took one page to explain. The thing to remember is that just because one subject took five times as many pages to explain, there will not necessarily be five times the number of questions on that subject. Here is some more specific advice on what to study:

1) **terms**—go through the glossary carefully. Make sure you can tell the difference between closely related terms.

2) **court decisions**—our textbooks are not law books, so there are not too many. But you should know what the issue was, the decision, why this was important, what effect it had on the industry, and approximately when it took place.

3) **NAIC model laws and regulations**—The actual laws and regulations appear as appendices are helpful, but we test on the text, not the appendices (although if something is not clear in the text, certainly use the appendices to clarify it—we do!)

4) **laws, especially federal laws**—DEFRA, COBRA, ERISA, OBRA-90, the HMO Act of 1973, etc.

5) **numbers**—Numbers appear in both the text and the charts. We do not expect you to memorize exact numbers, and there is no point in doing so since they change constantly. But we do expect you to have some idea of the magnitude—especially for comparison purposes—of certain key numbers. How many people are covered by individual health insurance? What percent of the population is that? Is this percent growing, shrinking, or stable? If the number is changing, how fast? This issue is covered in more detail in the following section, "Study Hints for HIAA Examinations."

6) **dates**—Dates and periods of time are important, especially when the payment of a claim hinges on a series of critical dates. However, as with numbers, you need dates as reference points for comparison. Dates also tell you the sequence of events, which is important for cause and effect. For some of the numbers in the text and charts, the date is important—how current is the data? Is it likely to be much different today? How fast are changes taking place?

7) **important topics that appear over and over again in different contexts**—HMOs, Medicare, federal and state regulations, different points of view (consumer, provider, payer).

8) **anything in the text with bullet points, multiple parts, multiple reasons**—this is a multiple choice test after all!

STUDY HINTS FOR HIAA EXAMINATIONS

This section explains HIAA testing procedures, dispels some of the misconceptions that may have developed concerning our exams, answers common questions, and gives a systematic explanation of the types of questions on the exams.

Can I rely on my experience alone to pass the exam?

Not necessarily. The HIAA textbooks reflect industry practices as a whole. Your experience might be with a company that departs from industry experience in one or more areas—and you might not even be aware of it. Another problem might be that your knowledge of a particular area is much deeper than the coverage given to that area in our textbook. This problem is covered in some detail in another part of this section, "Why do you have such tricky questions?"

Can I get answer keys to past exams, or to an exam I just took?

No. We have two main reasons: first, our courses qualify for continuing education credits in all but one of the states that offer such credits. Each state insurance department sets its own rules for granting credit. Many states have a requirement that answers are not to be given out to students—ever. So giving out answer keys would jeopardize our accreditation.

Secondly, our education committee and exam sub-committee have always advised against distributing answer keys. They believe that some students would be tempted to study only the old exams and ignore the textbooks as a short cut. (See section on "Should we use past exams as study aids?")

However, if there is a particular question, which, after deep reflection and thorough consultation with others, including your company Education Correspondent, still is completely baffling, you may call us and we will direct you to the page reference for an exam question. With thousands of students involved in each exam, this should obviously be a rare exception.

After my exam I checked my answers in the textbook, and I think one question had two answers that were correct (or no correct answers!). What do I do?

Again, the first step is to talk to others in your company who took that exam, or to your Education Correspondent. If you *still* think the exam is mistaken (no answer is correct, or two or more answers are correct), then you can formally challenge the question. Your challenge must be in writing, submitted through your Education Correspondent, and must reach HIAA by 4:30 PM Eastern time the next business day following the exam in question.

Make sure you give the name of the exam, the question number, and the reason you think the question is wrong (as well as your own name and your company, and the company address). All written challenges receive a written reply.

Occasionally we do eliminate certain questions from the scoring. But the time limit is important, since the exam grading and reporting process is both long and complicated. We cannot delay processing longer than necessary.

Please do not send in a challenge that simply proves that one of the choices is, in fact, a correct answer! Every question has a correct answer, and we already know which one it is!

Why are there so many questions about history?

This becomes almost a philosophical question, since in a sense everything is "history": Medicare, TEFRA, all regulations, etc. However, in a narrow sense there are some "history" questions, but statistically there are very few. Also please notice that some of the "history" questions are only superficially about a historical topic and are really asking something else altogether.

Is there a hidden pattern to the answers?

Definitely not! Our computer randomly arranges the answers within each question and thus also randomly decides the order of answers in the exam. The computer does this each time we make up an exam. For example, a certain question might have its answers arranged one way in spring 1991, and when the question appeared again in spring 1994, its answers would be in a different order. We do have an exception to this: answers that are numbers (dollars, numbers of days, etc.) or dates are always arranged in order from small/early to large/late ($50, $75, $100, $500 or May 1, May 9, May 31, June 1). By putting these answers in order, we alter the random order generated by the computer—we may, for example, change a correct answer in a question about dates from A to C. These changes usually cancel each other out—if we change one answer from A to C, another will be changed from C to A, etc. We do, however, keep an eye on the spread of A's, B's, C's, and D's: theoretically the computer could randomly generate a test that had all A's. That would be distracting to even the best students, and of course we would not allow that to happen. In fact, we do have guidelines for how many A's, B's, C's, and D's are allowed, but it is extremely rare for the computer to generate a spread of answers outside these guidelines.

Why do you ask questions about 'how many' of something there is when the number in the textbook is probably out of date? Should we be expected to memorize exact numbers?

Any question that deals with 'how many' is simply looking for an order of magnitude—a general idea of how many of something there is. Certainly you should have some idea of how many people are uninsured, how many health insurance companies there are, how many people have a certain kind of health insurance, and other useful numbers.

When we ask this type of question the "wrong" answers are very far from the "right" answer. We don't expect you to know exactly (no one does!) how many people are covered by managed care. But we do expect you to be able to make an estimate within 10 million or so. The wide margin also accounts for any recent changes.

For example, if we asked "How many members does the HIAA have?" we would never offer a set of answers like this:

A. 243.	But we might offer these:	A. 23.
B. 256.		B. 256
C. 265.		C. 1,817
D. 274		D. 245,768.

Why do you have such tricky questions?

None of our questions is intended to be "tricky." Each question is very straightforward, and it is a mistake to second- or third-guess it. But there are several considerations you should be aware of. This is a long answer, but an important one!

First, each question should be taken on its own terms, and at the level of sophistication with which it was treated in the textbook. Take a question about Medicare, for example. Our textbooks discuss Medicare, usually in connection with some other concept (like coordination of benefits, or its effect on long-term care insurance). But our textbooks do not pretend to be manuals detailing every nuance of Medicare regulations. Someone taking one of our exams who has worked with Medicare for many years should have a knowledge of Medicare that goes far beyond our textbooks and exam questions. Therefore an exam question which has simply "Part B of Medicare covers purchase or rental of certain medical equipment," as an answer to a question may be not quite true to an expert in the subject—the expert may begin to think of all sorts of exceptions and qualifications. That is the wrong approach—do not take a question on your terms, but on its own terms, and those of the textbook.

Let's use a non-insurance example of "relative truth":

Where is the National Geographic Society located?

A. Washington DC.
B. Berlin.
C. Katmandu.
D. Steve's backyard.

Assuming you are taking a US test on geography, the context should give you the answer: Washington DC. But what if you were taking the same test and were German, and in fact there was a German counterpart organization in Berlin whose name in translation was "National Geographic Society," or what if you had lived in Katmandu and realized that the National Geographic Society had a research office there? Or what if you knew Steve, and realized that yes, behind his house in Gaithersburg Maryland were the main administrative offices of the National Geographic Society? None of these things should matter in the context of the question: the German, the Nepalese, and Steve's friend should all realize that this question is being asked of thousands of other people who do not share their specialized knowledge and yet are expected to select a "correct" answer. Their specialized knowledge, while useful in other contexts, is irrelevant here. And, of course there is a perfectly acceptable alternative: Washington DC.

Or, to take another question:

Where is the Pentagon located?

A. South Arlington.
B. Washington DC.
C. Langley.
D. Prince George's County.

Any resident of Washington would have no trouble in selecting A as the correct answer. Someone who had never visited Washington would be stumped. But what if we altered the question:

Where is the Pentagon located?

A. Washington DC.
B. Baltimore.
C. Richmond.
D. Annapolis.

Clearly a "wrong" answer is now "right!" It's all relative! If you return from Europe and immigration in New York asks you where you live, and you answer "Chicago," even though you live in the suburb of Oak Park, clearly you are not lying to the official—you are just gearing your answer to his frame of reference. And that is what we expect you to do on HIAA exams.

A similar situation arises in questions where the "right" answer is demonstrably "wrong." In a previous example, it was implied that HIAA has 256 members. Possibly no one really knows, on a given day, exactly how many members there are. Members join and leave on a regular basis. What are the rules for judging membership: announcement of joining or leaving? Paying dues? When does membership expire—midnight of a certain day, or noon? The closer you are to any situation, the more complicated it is. But luckily none of this matters! The exact number doesn't matter—the order of magnitude does. If, on test day, the HIAA actually had, according to the best available records, 261 members instead of 256, 256 would still be the best answer if the other choices were 23, 1817, and 245,768.

The second part to the question of "trickiness" has to do with the construction of multiple choice questions. As in the examples above, any question can be made easy or hard depending on the level of the answer expected. Even "What is your name?" might have a vast range of possible right answers, depending on the circumstances and who is asking the question. When we look for distracters, or "wrong" answers, we can use several possibilities:

1) the "right" answer, but with some essential change. The key word here is "essential;" something that makes this choice wrong in its very essence, not just in matter of degree.

2) a "wrong" answer that was discussed in the text. One past question dealt with "advantages to employers;" the text also listed "advantages to employees." By offering a "wrong" choice that was an advantage to an employee, and not to an employer, we suspected (correctly) that some students would not know the difference.

3) a "wrong" answer that "sounds" good, and even exists, but is wrong in this context. "DEFRA" should ring a bell with almost all students—the question is, which bell? "Canadian companies must submit their financial records to regulatory authorities on the feast of St. Jean Baptiste" is pure fancy. Yet it has a Canadian ring to it; after all, isn't the feast of St. Jean a holiday in Quebec? It's even in June!

4) a total nonsense answer. Again, it sounds good, but there is no such thing. For example "Schedule ZOO-3045 is used to report investment income on the annual statement of health insurance companies."

Are there any hints in the way a question is worded?

Be careful of wording and read carefully! Questions that begin with a general statement like "Premiums are. . ." or "An experience refund is. . ." mean all premiums and all experience refunds—in general. A general statement is true about all members of that class: for example, these statements about cats:

"A cat is an animal." "Cats are animals."

Not some cats, or only at certain times: these are general statements, which are always true. Other times questions will explicitly say "always" and "never."

Other questions hedge by saying "Many companies. . . ." or "In some cases. . ." This is used quite often in the textbooks, since they are trying to describe general industry practice, not necessarily what every company does. Usually the text will say something like "Many companies do X, Y, and Z." The exam question might ask,

Many companies do

    A. X.
    B. K.
    C. Q.
    D. R.

K, Q, and R were never mentioned in the text; maybe some companies do them. But clearly the answer is X.

Be careful of words like "help." There is a world of difference between "This piece completes the puzzle," and "This piece helps to complete the puzzle." In the first case, the puzzle is definitely complete; in the second, it may or may not be complete—we don't know.

"Can," "may" and other such words are also something to look for. "Cats may weigh over 20 pounds" does not mean that all cats weigh over 20 pounds, or even that any cat in existence at this moment weighs over 20 pounds.

Be careful of substituting an option for an obligation:

"A person caught littering will be fined $50 or sentenced to one day in jail." A question about this statement might be:

    What is the penalty for littering?

        A. A fine of $50 or one day in jail.
        B. A fine of $50.
        C. One day in jail.
        D. A fine of $50 and one day in jail.

Only answer A is possible. Answer B or C would mean that either the fine or the jail term would always be the punishment, and the other option would not be a possibility, when in fact it would. Answer D is also not possible; both cannot be true at the same time.

On the other hand, you should never use grammatical hints to guess at the right answer. We try to make sure questions are phrased in such a way as to eliminate this possibility, by using "a(n)" if some answers begin with a vowel and some with a consonant sound, and by using both forms of the verb if an answer could be singular or plural. This is often the case in the multiple option questions, which have a specific grammatical disclaimer in the instructions. If a question is phrased in the singular, it does not necessarily mean only one answer is possible, and vice versa.

Why do you force us to memorize the textbook? (50% of students) vs. Why isn't the answer in the textbook—are we supposed to make assumptions, inferences, and generalizations? (the other 50% of students!)

In general, questions tend to stick to the language in the textbook. This is not an effort to make students memorize the book, but simply because the textbook usually says it the best way. But many questions paraphrase the textbook, and some *do* ask for assumptions, inferences, generalizations, and judgments. The answers are still "in the book" in the sense that a reasonable person could be expected to consistently come up with the "correct" answer.

We are caught between two conflicting points of view, as are all test-makers. A test must measure what it's supposed to measure to be valid. HIAA tests knowledge of life and health insurance, and more specifically, our textbooks. We do our best to make sure the textbooks reflect the latest developments in the industry.

Beyond that, every test must also measure many skills. For example, our tests are in English. So they also measure reading speed, reading comprehension, and vocabulary. This could be a problem for some people—and not just those whose native language is not English! Math questions also involve a knowledge of arithmetic. Even filling in the circles on the answer sheet is a skill, and thus is being tested.

Should we use past exams as study aids?

Yes and no. Certainly past exams are good samples of the types of questions you can expect. However you will be sadly disappointed if you expect to see the identical questions on a future exam!! Approximately half the questions on any given exam are changed before they are used again. These modified questions then go back into our database of questions. Some of the changes may be slight—so slight you don't notice them—but most of the time they affect the answer significantly. Negative questions can turn into positive questions, and vice versa. The insertion of a word like "not" or "all" can make a correct answer wrong or a wrong answer right. What was once the correct answer can change completely (more than one right answer is usually possible, after all) and the wrong choices which seemed so silly and obvious on a past exam can be modified so that only the very best students will be able to identify them as "wrong."

Generally 20–25% of the questions on any given exam are completely new. Another 50% or so are modified questions—they have appeared in some form in past exams (during the last 15 years!) but have now been changed. That leaves 25–30% of the questions that, in fact, have appeared in identical form on past exams. But which past exam? A question could have appeared in spring 1984. . . . or fall 1989 . . . or . . . . Furthermore, have you ever wondered why identical questions continue to appear? There is only one answer: they are effective questions! And effective questions separate knowledgeable students from ones who do not know the subject thoroughly.

It is a questionable use of time to go through 15 years' worth of 100-question exams in hopes of memorizing the 25–30% of repeat questions—without even knowing which ones they are and without answer keys! It would be far better to read the textbook thoroughly.

I don't have access to old exams!! What are the questions like?

Each Study Manual has sample questions, with answers, at the back.

Chapter 1

MANAGED CARE AND THE RESTRUCTURING OF HEALTH CARE FOR AMERICANS IN THE 1990s: AN OVERVIEW

■ Key Terms

Employer coalitions

Employment Retirement Income Security Act (ERISA)

Health Insurance Portability and Accountability Act (HIPAA)

Managed care "lite"

Managed indemnity

Market consolidation

Medicaid managed care

Medical Savings Accounts (MSAs)

Medicare managed care

Open-access plans

Patient Protection Act

Point-of-service (POS) plans

Preferred provider organization (PPO) plans

Provider-sponsored MCO

1. How has the market presence of managed care organizations (MCOs) changed in the last decade?

   Growing a 18.7% annually

2. What are two alternate early names for health maintenance organizations (HMOs)?

   prepaid practice plans   alternative delivery systems

3. How did HMOs succeed, or even exist, initially?

   Supported federal grants + regulatory protection

4. What are three reasons that managed care's cost controls have accelerated the movement away from traditional indemnity insurance?

   Pg 4   *reduced the utilization of hospitals and ancillary services, decreased excess testing, and brought health inflation rates below the consumer price index.*

5. How many U.S. cities have greater than 50% managed care enrollment? What are two reasons for this?   *10 cities*   *① gov't workers concentration ② state capitals in 3 cities*

6. Why is Blue Cross/Blue Shield, one of the nation's leading indemnity insurers, only a 2nd tier managed care player in many markets?

   Hesitancy to enter the managed care market

7. Give some examples of markets where top MCOs are not national firms.

   Harris Methodist Dallas Fort Worth
   Kaiser, Pacificare/FHP, and Foundation Health Calif

8. What is the typical MCO distribution of market share in large metropolitan markets (more than one million population)?

   leader holds a 38% market share
   number 2 plans holds a 21% share
   number 3 plan holds a 12% share
   remaining 29% is divided among 15-20 MCOs

9. In mid-sized (250,000 to one million population) and small (under 250,000) markets?

   More concentrated   least competitive
   leader commanding 53% share   leader 69% share

10. Why did MCO enrollment fall in some markets in 1996?

    reflects those consumers who are "buying up" to obtain greater access and choice by switching to preferred provider organizations

11. What should MCOs do to improve their public image? *become better citizens show they care about more than profits offer something special managing care*

12. What are provider-sponsored MCOs and why are they gaining market share in some areas? *physicians + Hospitals sponsored employers are looking*

13. What percent of U.S. workers with health insurance now receive their coverage through an MCO? *80%*

14. What is managed care "lite"? *Between Hmos + traditional plans*

15. What reforms did Congress enact in 1997 to change Medicare-related managed care? *medicare - related managed care reforms medicare Hmos raising the floor of medicare Hmo payments to $350 member/per month eliminating l'il req. creating PPO + PSO Options*

Pg 7

16. Why might these changes expand managed care in rural areas? *Because where medicare Hmo fees are below cost under the old scheme of medicare HMO payments*

17. Why are states implementing managed care programs for Medicaid beneficiaries? *Because of the predictable costs of managed care programs*

18. What are employer coalitions and how might they affect the future of health care?

19. What are two ways that ERISA protections of employer sponsored plans have been eroded? *Erisa plans need to provide "parity" between mental health and other health plans Courts weakened "Any willing provider" law forcing employer self funded plans to open pharmacy networks to compete w pharmacies*

20. What are two strategies HMOs are using to boost market share? *offer a more varied portfolio product lines reshaped*

21. According to recent estimates, what portion of the market did POS plans have in 1997?

20.1 %

22. Why is the POS form of "lite" managed care becoming so popular?

enrollers are given more choices + partial coverage if they use out of network health services

23. How do open-access plans differ from POS plans?

offer lower-cost alternative to POS plans with greater access to specialists
patients are allowed to bypass gatekeeper w/in MCO network

24. Why are PPOs popular among fee-for-service providers?

because there are few limitations on the amount of services they can provide but must keep their charges low

25. Typically, how much more do managed indemnity plans cost than MCOs in the same market?

Indemnity plans are priced 25-40% higher than MCO's in the same market

26. What are two restrictions managed indemnity plans require?

Prior authorization for expensive services
may deny claims for services that the plans consider medically unnecessary

27. How do Medical Savings Accounts work?

combine a high deductible ins policy with a savings account. The savings from a higher deductible goes to an MSA account to cover routine medical expenses, while the high deductible ins plan covers exp that exceed the deductible

28. What are six types of laws states have passed to control or regulate MCOs?

1. providers who are under incentive clauses to limit care must disclose financial conflicts of interest 2 gag rules, which prohibit physicians from criticizing plans or fully informing patients about treatments, are prohibited 3 physician, hospital, chiropractors, pharmac and others cannot be shut out of hmo contracts if the providers are willing to accept hmo prices and terms (any willing provider law) 4 consumers are guaranteed choice of plan options 5 in Texas, managed care plans are specifically identified as potentially liable for d

29. What has been the recent relationship between MCO enrollment and profit?

Enrollment rose and profits declined

30. What are some benefits for MCOs to consolidate?

market domination

31. What are eight things MCOs must consider doing to survive in the increasingly competitive health care market?

① Be Consumer Driven
Simplify access + increase choices
Remain Price Competitive
Promote Clinically Efficient Processes
Reduce Overhead
Establish Provider alliances
Demonstrate Value to Purchasers
Accept accountability

...s of treatment on 6 HMO's and insurers cannot arbitrarily drop a provider from the network without a fair hearing (ie due process)

Chapter 2

MANAGED CARE AND THE REGULATORY ARENA

■ Key Terms

Accreditation

Appeals and grievance systems

The "business of insurance"

Capitation

Confidentiality clauses

Consolidated Licensure for Entities Assuming Risk (CLEAR)

Emergency Medical Treatment and Active Labor Act (EMTALA)

ERISA preemption

Federal HMO Act

Limits of state regulatory authority

Mandated benefits

Maryland Health Care Access and Cost Commission's HMO Quality Report Card

Mental health parity

National Association of Insurance Commissioners (NAIC)

NCQA's *Health Plan Employer Data and Information Set* (HEDIS)

Payer and medical director liability

Provider networks

Provider-sponsored networks (PSNs)

Risk-bearing entities

Utilization review

Utilization Review and Accreditation Commission (URAC)

Vertical/horizontal industry regulation

Virginia Bureau of Insurance (VBOI)

1. What is horizontal regulation? Give two examples.

reaches across the boundaries of all industries
OSHA EEOC EPA CPSC

2. What is vertical regulation? Give two examples.

focuses solely on their industry FCC for radio + tv
FDA - manufacture + distribution of drugs

3. How do vertical and horizontal regulation affect the insurance industry? Discuss both the state and federal governments.

Have Both
The states regulated the business of insurance while most of the other employee benefits fell to the US Dept of Labor - State pushed back

4. What is the NAIC?

National Association of Insurance - the oldest association of state officials

5. What is the significance of the McCarran-Ferguson Act?

act which reserved to the states the regulation of the "business of insurance"

6. What three questions has the U.S. Supreme Court outlined to help determine whether an activity is the business of insurance, and therefore subject only to state control, or the business of insurers or some other realm subject to federal regulation as well? Are the tests determinative?

• Does the activity have "the effect of transferring or spreading a policy holder's risk?
• Is the activity "an integral part of the policy relationship between the insurer and the insured?"
• Is the activity "limited to entities within

7. Why is determining the boundary between state and federal regulation of MCOs so complex and diverse?

ERISA is federal   Insurance is state
must be clear and it won't always

8. What is the VBOI and why is it significant?

VBOI Virginia Bureau of Insurance
issued an administrative letter explaining that all capitation arrangements involved the transfer of risk and, thus, the business of insurance

3rd Party Administrators w/capitated arrangements are not subject to ERISA

Consolidated Licensure for Entities Assuming Risk

9. What is the NAIC's CLEAR project?

create a seamless licensure process for all entities assuming risk, no matter what the corporate structure of such entities

10. What are the two primary regulatory responses to health care provider organizations' requests that solvency requirements for PSNs be eased?

CAPITATION

State regulators allowed PSNs to assume risk from licensed health carriers without meeting HMO or insurer regulatory req Regulators are much less inclined to allow such unregulated risk assumption directly from employers

11. What information is it commonly believed that consumers lack regarding their health care plans?

How to access care, how physicians are paid, and how to "work" the system

12. Why do consumers need information and what information do they need?

price of health coverage is substantial and the consequences of poor quality are profound

Price

Quality

13. What two things do states generally require as far as carrier disclosure?

markers of health plan quality and uniformity of reporting methodology

14. What is HEDIS? Give an example of how it's been utilized.

Health Plan Employer Data and Information Set
Standardized reporting

15. What are "gag clauses" and what has the response been to their purported widespread use?

Prohibited physicians from fully apprising their patients of their treatment options
Legislature responded with a flurry of activity
40 states - limit gag clauses

16. What is accreditation and who accomplishes it?

minimum quality standards

accrediting institutions

17. Why is a uniform definition of "medical necessity" becoming increasingly important?

public confusion   boundry of health coverage vs clinical determination by the treating physician

18. Name five benefits that federal and state laws and regulations may require MCOs to provide.

*1 mammograms or Pap smears
3 treatment of certain ailments
4 minimum length of stay mother + newborn
5 minimum length of stay mastectomies*

19. What does the Mental Health Parity Act of 1996 require?

requires that group plans that provide medical and mental health coverage not impose more restrictive annual and lifetime dollar limits on mental health benefits than they do on medical benefit

20. What are two potential disadvantages to mandated benefits?

Plan solvency   Physician dominance of clinical decisions

21. What is one increasingly popular alternative to state legislatures mandating minimum benefits?

Use a process by which a commission, outside the normal legislative process, evaluates proposed mandates for clinical efficacy and economic impact

22. Why are "any willing provider" (AWP) laws proving to be controversial in managed care?

MCOs argue that an AWP law erodes their ability to manage the quality of the panel and negotiate discounts with providers

23. What is a mandatory POS law?

Plans are required to offer at least the employer a choice between a closed panel HMO and either a POS product or an indemnity product

24. What specialties are typically included in state direct access laws?

Obstetrics and gynecology, dermatology, chiropractic nurse practitioner

25. What is capitation?

Pay per member not service

26. What do MCOs argue in defense of capitation arrangements?

Capitated arrangements only affect over utilization not proper utilization

27. What percentage of physician groups report capitation compensation?

60%

28. What are some requirements that states are considering regarding capitation arrangements or bonus/withhold methodologies?

29. What is EMTALA and what does it require?

Emergency medical Treatment + Active Labor Act

30. How has the government responded to the policy arguments between MCOs and emergency rooms regarding emergency treatment of members?

31. What are three formulary restrictions currently in effect in or under consideration by various states?

32. What public laws and private agencies typically affect MCOs?

33. What are two approaches state laws take to improve MCO accountability for coverage decisions?

34. What is ERISA's limitation on MCO tort liability for ERISA plans?

35. What is *respondeat superior* and how does it apply to MCOs?

36. Why is the 1997 Texas law SB 386 potentially significant for MCOs?

37. Why is utilization review a relatively controversial topic in terms of health plan liability?

Chapter 3

MANAGED CARE AND THE CONSUMER

■ Key Terms

Agency for HealthCare Policy and Research (AHCPR)

Commonwealth Foundation Survey (1995)

Consumer protection laws

Foundation for Accountability (FACCT)

Health Insurance Portability and Accountability Act (HIPAA)

HEDIS data

Medical record confidentiality standards

National Association of Insurance Commissioners' (NAIC's) model acts

Polling data

President's Advisory Commission on Consumer Protection and Quality in the Health Care Industry

Consumer protection standards

State consumer protection laws

1. By the end of the 1980s, a popular belief emerged that health care costs no longer reflected economic reality. Why?

2. Why are some MCO cost control strategies, so important in curbing double digit health care inflation in the late 1980s, now seen in a negative light?

3. What did the Commonwealth Fund Foundation's 1995 survey show?

4. What did the 1997 Kaiser Family Foundation survey show?

5. What percentage of Americans favor a consumer or patients' bill of rights? How does that change if premiums change?

6. In general, what does the polling data show public opinion about the current managed care system to be?

7. How has media coverage affected managed care in the 1990s?

8. Name two examples of how normally business-friendly Republicans are supporting increased government oversight of health plans.

9. What percentage of Americans favor a law requiring health plans to provide information about operations, covered benefits, participating doctors, and grievance resolution procedures?

10. Typically, what do state managed care consumer protection laws require health plans to disclose?

11. Who typically uses the NCQA's HEDIS data?

12. What is FACCT and what does it do?

13. What is the standard consumer survey instrument for the industry and who developed it?

14. What has the Clinton administration done to address public concern over the security and confidentiality of medical records?

15. Name two states that mandate that health plans provide a POS option to enrollees.

16. The largest percentage of the public wants managed care regulated by

17. What does the 1996 New York consumer protection bill for managed care enrollees require?

18. How does New Jersey's HMO Consumer Bill of Rights differ?

19. What did California Governor Pete Wilson's 30-member Commission on Managed Care recommend in its January 1998 report?

20. Why is the May 1998 ruling of the Texas Attorney General significant?

21. What are the NAIC model acts?

22. What would be the advantages and disadvantages to federal consumer protection regulation?

23. What are the purposes and positive features of HIPAA?

24. What do the new internal Medicare regulations and Congress's Balanced Budget Act of 1997 changes require?

25. The President's Advisory Commission on Consumer Protection and Quality in the Health Care Industry issued a report in November 1997 recommending what "rights"?

26. What did President Clinton order in February 1998?

Chapter 4

MANAGED CARE AND PUBLIC AND PRIVATE PURCHASING GROUPS

■ Key Terms

Accreditation

Business groups/coalitions

Buyers Health Care Action Group (BHCAG) in Minneapolis

Coalition continuity

Collective purchasing

Community Health Purchasing Corporation in Des Moines, Iowa

Employer coalitions

Foundation for Accountability (FACCT)

Gateway Purchasing Association in St. Louis

Health Care Financing Administration (HFCA)

Health Insurance Plan of California (HIPC)

Joint Commission on Accreditation of Health Care Organizations (JCAHO)

Multiple Employer Trusts (METs)

Multiple Employer Welfare Association (MEWA)

National Business Coalition on Health (NBCH)

National Committee for Quality Assurance (NCQA)

Pacific Business Group on Health (PBGH)

Partnerships

Professional Standards Review Organizations (PSROs)

Quality monitoring

Small employer

Taft-Hartley Trusts

Tax Equity and Fiscal Responsibility Act of 1982 (TEFRA)

Washington Business Group on Health (WBGH)

1. What are PSROs and what do they do?

2. What management approaches have PSROs taken?

3. Why did large insurers begin incorporating utilization review into their own lines of business?

4. How do multisite employers sometimes handle health care expenses and management?

5. How can employers evaluate health plans?

6. What do most employers want to protect themselves against in their health plan contracts?

7. What are two benefits for large employers who self-insure or self-fund?

8. What is the Health Insurance Plan of California?

9. What is a collective purchasing arrangement and what is its goal?

10. What cities have established collective employer purchasing arrangements?

11. How are health benefit trusts typically organized?

12. What federal laws specifically mention health benefit trusts?

13. What are METs and MEWAs and what is their advantage?

14. What are Taft-Hartley trusts?

15. What do health plan marketing experts believe is the best way to reach future plan participants?

16. In smaller or rural communities, how can employers provide managed care benefits for their employees?

17. Why do employers and communities sometimes work together in the health care arena?

18. When did business and employer coalitions appear?

19. What is the current approach taken by employer coalitions?

20. Give two examples of national coalitions and a brief description of each.

21. Why is a coalition's size important?

22. Give two reasons why participation by a state employee benefit plan or Medicaid program enhances a coalition's impact.

23. What are Gateway Purchasing Association and Community Health Purchasing Corporation?

24. Typically, what activities do coalitions focus on?

25. Why must health care coalitions continue to re-evaluate themselves?

Chapter 5

THE FEDERAL EMPLOYEES HEALTH BENEFITS PROGRAM

■ Key Terms

Adjusted Community Rating (ACR)

Annual "open season"

Annuitants

Benefits Administration Letter

"Call Letter"

Cancellation, termination

Community rating

Community rating by class (CRC)

Complaints

Enrollment records

Enrollments, reconciliations, underpayments

Experience rating

Federal Acquisition Regulations (FAR)

Federal Employees Health Benefits (FEHB) Program

Federal Employees Health Benefits Acquisition Regulation (FEHBAR)

Headcount Report

Insurance officer

Office of Personnel Management (OPM)

Office of the Inspector General (OIG)

OPM Office of Retirement Programs

OPM Office of the Inspector General (IG)

Rate/benefit negotiations

Service charge

Similarly sized subscriber groups (SSSGs)

US Office of Personnel Management (OPM)

1. When was the Federal Employees Health Benefits (FEHB) Program established?

7-1-1960

2. How many enrollees does it currently have?

9.5 mill enrollees   350 carriers

3. Who administers the FEHB Program?

OPM

4. What three types of health plans does OPM contract for?

1 government wide 2 employee org sponsored by federal union
3. comprehensive medical plans

5. Under what laws does the FEHB Program exist and operate?

FEHB Act

6. When is the annual federal health benefits open season?

Nov DEC

7. Identify and explain the six major differences (besides size) between the FEHB Program and other employer-sponsored health programs.

Acceptance
Effective Dates
Enrollment records
Insurance Officer
Premiums
member lists

8. When is the OPM's Office of Insurance Program's "Call Letter" issued to participating carriers?

3/31

9. What are the deadlines for plans to submit proposed changes to OPM?

5/31

10. During what time period do OPM and the plans negotiate?

June through August

11. How are Annual Open Season dates announced?

Press release F

12. How do carriers market their plans to federal workers?

OPM issues Benefit Admin letter

13. How are enrollee complaints and disputes handled?

14. When can a carrier terminate a federal enrollee?

Can't

15. What is OPM's role in reconciling enrollment records?

16. What are Headcount Reports and when are they issued?

17. Why do underpayments typically occur in the FEHB Program?

18. Identify and describe three types of community rating used in the FEHB Program.

19. What is the OPM's contingency reserve?

20. What factors does OPM apply to determine the "service charge" or profit each experience-rated plan receives?

21. What costs are allowable under experience-rated plans?

22. Beginning in 1999, what is the government contribution toward the cost of health benefits under the FEHB Program?

23. What two types of audits are generally conducted for community-rated plans?

24. What are SSSGs?

25. What is a Certificate of Accurate Pricing?

26. What specific areas may be covered in an experience-rated plan audit?

Chapter 6

TRICARE: A MANAGED CARE OPTION

■ Key Terms

Department of Defense (DOD)

"Ghosts"

Medicare managed care demonstration
project

Military Treatment Facility (MTF)

TRICARE Extra

TRICARE Prime

TRICARE Standard

1. What is the DOD's primary health care mission?

[handwritten: 15 bill = 6/0]

2. What is the Defense Health Program's annual budget?

3. What are MTFs and approximately how many exist worldwide?

[handwritten: 115 hosp   470 clincs]

4. What were the DOD's purposes in launching TRICARE in 1993?

5. How does the DOD handle the fact that it lacks military-owned or -operated facilities that are geographically accessible to every beneficiary?

6. For how many, and to which, regions had DOD awarded TRICARE contracts as of June 1998?

7. How are the three TRICARE options characterized?

[handwritten: Prime / Extra / Standard]

8. Under which TRICARE Option do beneficiaries not typically pay copayments or deductibles?

[handwritten: PRIME]

9. What are "ghosts" and why is the DOD concerned about them?

10. What shift does the DOD project in numbers of individuals eligible for military health care benefits?

11. What amendment did the Balanced Budget Act of 1997 include that has significance for DOD and Medicare?

Chapter 7

MANAGED CARE IN MEDICARE

■ Key Terms

Adjusted average per capita cost (AAPCC)

"Age-ins"

Amount per member, per month

Annual audit

Balanced Budget Act of 1997 (BBA '97)

Beneficiary eligibility

Competitive Medical Plan

Coordinated care plans

Disclosure rules

Encounter data

Enrollment, disenrollment

Foundation for Accountability (FACCT)

Health Care Prepayment Plan (HCPP)

Medical Savings Account (MSA)

Medicare+Choice

Payment rates

Plan user fees

Private fee-for-service plans

Provider participation

Public Law 105-33, the BBA '97

Quality requirements

Religious, fraternal benefit society plans

Section 1876 contracts

Special Information Campaign

1. The HCFA is the _____*largest*_____ purchaser of managed care in the country.

2. What things does HCFA evaluate in the process of contracting with risk plans?

3. What is the AAPCC?

4. The BBA '97created what important program?

   Medicare Part C

5. Identify and describe the three types of entities that may be granted contracts by HCFA under Medicare+Choice.

6. As of what date do existing Section 1876 contracts terminate?

   Jan 1, 1999

7. As of January 1, 1999, what are the limits on DHHS's authority to contract with HCPPs?

   unions

8. What beneficiaries are entitled to enroll in a Medicare+Choice plan?

9. What does Medicare assume about newly eligible enrollees who do not select a Medicare+Choice plan?

10. How does the new law treat beneficiaries enrolled in an 1876 plan as of December 31, 1998?

11. After January 1, 2003, what time frame do beneficiaries have to change enrollment options?

12. What are three possible exceptions to that time frame?

13. Under what circumstances may a Medicare+Choice plan disenroll a Medicare beneficiary?

14. What new Medicare benefits does the BBA '97 provide for?

15. What must Medicare+Choice plans disclose to enrollees?

16. What information may enrollees request plans to provide?

17. What non-network provider services must Medicare+Choice plans cover?

18. How does Medicare+Choice define "emergency medical condition"?

19. What does BBA '97's "conscience protection" clause provide?

20. What rules does Medicare have to ensure that incentives to discourage unnecessary services do not jeopardize quality?

21. In general, how are the Medicare capitation rates determined?

22. What must all Medicare+Choice plans have submitted by May 1998?

23. What tools do HCFA and DHHS use to monitor and ensure quality of care?

24. Identify and describe the four additional reporting requirements that Medicare+Choice plans must meet.

Chapter 8

STATE GOVERNMENT AS PURCHASER OF MANAGED CARE

■ Key Terms

"Auto enrollments"

Consumer satisfaction surveys

"Dual-eligibles"

External reviews

Incentives and sanctions

Joint Commission on Accreditation of
Healthcare Organizations (JCAHO)

Medicaid HEDIS data set

National Committee for Quality Assurance
(NCQA)

Peer Review Organizations (PROs)

Primary Care Case Manager (PCCM)

Purchasing for value

Quality improvement studies

"Safety net"

Section 1115 waiver

Section 1915(b) of the Social Security Act

1. What are the two major population groups for which states purchase health care?

[handwritten: State emp   medicade beneficiaries]

2. What did Section 1915(b) of the Social Security Act, passed by Congress in 1981, authorize DHHS to do?

3. How does a PCCM differ from a managed care plan?

4. What three things are believed to have fueled the Medicaid managed care explosion of the 1990s?

5. Typically, what four low-income populations does Medicaid cover?

6. What was the percentage increase in Medicaid enrollment between 1992 and 1996?

7. Where is most Medicaid enrollment growth expected in the near future?

8. What did BBA '97 do for Medicaid managed care?

9. What are the disadvantages of PCCMs versus plans?

10. What are the positives and negatives of carve-outs and special purpose plans?

11. Identify and describe the five tools states typically use to influence the quality of medical care.

12. Before the growth of managed care, where did the Medicaid and medically indigent populations usually go for medical services?

13. What does it mean to "risk-adjust" capitation rates?

14. What can states do to minimize compliance burdens and maximize analysis and evaluation of plans?

15. What two states have made attempts to standardize their Medicaid contract specifications and how have they done so?

Chapter 9

PHARMACY BENEFIT MANAGEMENT PROGRAMS

■ Key Terms

"Carve-outs"

Average wholesale price (AWP)

Benefit design references

Clinical and administrative edits

Clinical management programs

Closed formulary

Customer service program

Disease management program

Dispensing fee

Drug benefit management

Drug use evaluation (DUE)

Drug utilization reports

Drug utilization review (DUR)

Electronic claims processing

Generic drugs

Integrated pharmacy programs

Mail service pharmacy

NCQA/HEDIS

Open formulary

Patient profiling

"Pay for Performance" program

Pharmaceutical manufacturer discounts/rebates

Pharmacy and Therapeutic (P and T) Committee

Pharmacy benefit management company (PBM)

Pharmacy benefit plan reporting

Pharmacy care program

Pharmacy networks

Preferred formulary

Prior authentication

Processing performance standards

Provider profiling

Therapeutic interchange

Treatment guidelines

Universal Claim Form (UCF)

1. Name three reasons insurers began to consider new ways to manage prescription drug benefits in the 1980s.

2. Initially, how were pharmacy claims processed?

3. What is the UCF?

4. What are three characteristics of today's prescription drug programs?

5. What clinical management programs do MCOs frequently use to control costs and improve patient care?

6. What do MCOs do in using the restricted network approach for pharmacy networks?

7. What are the advantages to a restricted network?

8. What is the typical range for AWP discounts in pharmacy networks today?

9. Why is online, real-time claim processing an improvement over paper or batch processing?

10. What are the 13 administrative and 12 clinical edits frequently used in electronic claim processing?

myd $0.20

11. Administrative fees for high-volume carriers or plans are commonly in the _____ per claim range.

12. What are the performance standards for today's prescription plans?

13. Identify ten common exclusions in pharmaceutical benefit designs.

14. Approximately what percentage of prescriptions filled annually go through mail service programs?

15. What are the advantages and disadvantages of mail service programs to MCOs?

16. What are typical performance standards expected of an MCO's service representatives?

17. What is a P & T committee and what are its mission and role?

18. What is a drug formulary? What is its purpose?

19. What criteria are used to evaluate drugs for formulary inclusion?

20. Identify and describe the three basic types of drug formularies.

21. Distinguish between positive and negative closed formularies.

22. Besides cost savings, what is another common result of therapeutic interchanges?

23. What requirements are often included for an MCO to get pharmaceutical manufacturer discounts or rebates?

24. Why are treatment guidelines generally acceptable to physicians?

25. What drugs are typically designated for prior authorization?

26. What steps are usually taken to establish a DUR or DUE program?

27. Identify and describe the three common types of DURs.

28. What components do most disease management programs include?

29. Typically, what disease states might be addressed by such a program?

30. How often are disease management program outcomes measured?

31. Name and describe the three categories of medication education typically used by MCOs and the subcontractors.

32. How is pharmacy benefit reporting generally available today?

33. What indicators do most pharmacy program managers continually review?

34. Why is patient profiling important?

35. How are outcomes of disease management programs measured?

36. Identify 12 pharmacy-specific indicators the NCQA uses to measure effectiveness of care.

37. Describe the role of and services offered by PBMs.

38. What is the recent controversy surrounding ownership of PBMs?

39. What is the effect of carving-out prescription drug benefits rather than having integrated pharmacy programs?

Chapter 10

MANAGED DENTAL CARE

■ Key Terms

Alternate treatment

Copayment

Critical mass

Dental health maintenance organization
(DHMO)

Dental practice management company
(DPMC)

Dental preferred provider organization
(DPPO)

Dental service organization (DSO)

Electronic submission

Gatekeeper

Least expensive alternate treatment (LEAT)

National Association of Dental Plans
(NADP)

Network model

Quality of care measurement

Staff model

Utilization

1. What combination of factors is enabling people to keep their teeth longer?

2. Why will dentist availability be a challenge for managed care plans in the near future?

3. According to NADP, what percent of the population is covered by dental plans?

45

4. Why is dental insurance not insurance in the classic sense?

5. Why do dental patients seldom self-refer to dental specialists?

6. Currently, what percent of dentists participate in managed care?

7. To what two diseases does dental care primarily apply?

8. What is LEAT and how is it used?

9. What if a patient wants a more expensive alternative treatment than one the dental plan will cover?

they pay

10. Identify and describe the five basic models most dental managed care plans follow.

11. Which model is most commonly used in conjunction with a dental HMO or PPO? *Network*

12. What percentage of dentists participated in dental HMOs in 1997?

13. Identify four areas in which dental PPOs have advantages over HMOs.

14. Typically, managed care requires a comprehensive information system. What specific data requirements must a dental plan include?

15. Why will group practices become the backbone of dental managed care?

16. What are "retentions" and why are excessive retentions troublesome?

17. How many dental schools, and how many first year students, were there in America in 1998? Why are these numbers significant?

18. What three factors make it more difficult to recruit dentists to participate in managed care plans?

19. Where are dental care's largest costs incurred?

20. What are DMPCs?

21. Why is electronic data interchange important to dental managed care?

Chapter 11

BEHAVIORAL HEALTH PROBLEMS

■ Key Terms

Accreditation

Cottage industry

Integrated delivery system

Outcome studies

Practice guidelines

Provider profiles

System delivery

Treatment options

Vertically integrated network

1. Why do some providers oppose managed care?

2. Identify and describe the five specific obstacles that complicate behavioral health managed care.

3. Why are confidentiality issues so important to behavioral health services?

4. What is one of the biggest challenges facing the establishment of behavioral managed care?

5. What ten components are usually considered part of a full continuum for behavioral health?

6. What are two approaches providers can take to integrate or expand services?

7. What disciplines must behavioral health providers demonstrate expertise in to succeed in managed care?

8. What are provider profiles and why are they important to managed care?

9. Why is it important that the NCQA scores MCOs on how well they promote provider participation in the development of practice guidelines?

10. What seven areas does the NCQA typically measure in accrediting behavioral health care organizations?

Chapter 12

VISION CARE PROGRAMS

■ Key Terms

Capitated carve-out

Disease detection

Eyewear fabrication

Fashion component

Management services

Medical eye care

Opthamologist

Optician

Optometrist

Routine vision care

Surgical eye care

Unique service

Vision benefit managers (VBMs)

Vision care

1. What percentage of Americans are currently in need of vision correction?

    60% 10

2. Why is the number of people in need of corrective eyewear expected to grow by over a million people a year until 2011?

3. Why is vision care considered unique among health care services?

4. How can routine eye exams aid in early disease detection?

5. How important did 61% of surveyed adults feel that vision care is?

6. Why are vision care benefits increasingly popular with MCO plan managers?

7. What does routine vision care typically include?

8. What level of vision care is usually included in managed care plans?

9. What does that coverage include?

10. What do surgical eyecare services almost always require in the managed care environment?

11. What are VBMs and what do they do?

12. In what two ways do VBMs enhance MCOs?

13. How are VBM delegations typically structured?

14. How do opticians, optometrists, and opthamologists differ?

15. Why do many MCOs and VBMs require use of a designated ophthalmic laboratory?

Chapter 13

MANAGED CARE AND THE PHYSICIAN TODAY

■ Key Terms

Academic Health Centers (AHCs)

Core attitudes

Coverage exclusions

Different orientations

"Free-riders"

Market-driven arrangements

Partner with competitors

Physician buy-in

Reward positive performance

Risk selection

Tangible value

Target oversight

Three-tier system

Two-tier system

Values contrasts

1. What is the primary reason relations between MCOs and physicians became adversarial?

2. What is an "open-panel network"?

3. What is the difference between the two-tier system and the three-tier system and which approach is more common?

4. Identify three underlying values that physicians have that are in contrast to MCOs.

5. Why do MCOs really have two customers?

6. Identify five ways in which physicians' and MCOs' core attitudes and behavior patterns differ.

7. How do age variances among physicians affect their attitudes toward managed care?

8. How do the unique features of managed care interfere with the competitive, free-market strategies of other businesses?

9. How does the current market approach limit the MCO's ability to distinguish itself in the marketplace?

10. Why is the standardization physicians want problematic for MCOs?

11. What are some examples of MCO innovation?

12. What are "Free-Riders"?

13. Identify two reasons why specialists might be particularly resistant to or resentful of managed care.

14. What are AHCs and how are they affected by managed care?

15. Why are coverage exclusions problematic for physicians?

16. Identify and describe 10 steps that MCOs can take to build better relationships with doctors and produce a better managed care product.

17. What is the most effective way for MCOs to educate physicians?

18. Where is it most important to treat physicians fairly and consistently?

19. In what three areas are MCOs positioned to provide tangible value to physicians?

20. Why is the three-tier system emerging in the health care marketplace?

21. Where have the bulk of newer provider-based organizations such as IPAs and IDSs developed?

Chapter 14

MEASURING AND MANAGING THE QUALITY OF CARE

■ Key Terms

Accreditation

Clinical practice guidelines

Confidentiality

Consumer Assessment of Health Plans
Surveys (CAHPS)

Data management

Disease management

Disease-specific questionnaires

Ethical, medico-legal considerations

Evidence-based medicine

FDA Modernization Act of 1997

Health continuum model

Health management

Health Plan Employer Data and
Information Set (HEDIS)

Health risk assessments (HRAs)

Intervention modalities

JCAHO

NCQA

Patient-centered outcomes measurement

Population-based geographic analysis

Practice guidelines

Prevention programs

Primary prevention

Quality indicators

Quality of life and functional status
assessment

Reporting results

Secondary prevention

Short Form 36 Health Survey

Small-area variation analysis

Total quality management/continuous
quality improvement (TQM/CQI)

Utilization management (UM)

Wellness programs

1. What are three primary distinctions between traditional insurance and managed care?

2. What was the earliest and most prevalent form of health care control?

3. What message did early managed care fail to get out to consumers?

4. What four factors complicate MCOs' efforts to balance cost and quality in health care?

5. What did HMOs do initially to help contain costs?

6. Why is improving members' health important to MCOs?

7. What is the average turnover rate in managed care?

8. Identify three reasons an HMO should still invest in prevention.

9. Why do employers want a healthier workforce?

10. What new innovations and technologies can help MCOs achieve a needed paradigm shift?

11. How can MCOs use population-based geographic claims data?

12. Why are practice guidelines important for managed care?

13. What breakdown categories of facts can be useful in analyzing large data sets?

14. Why do MCOs need to demonstrate results?

15. What is a primary indicator of quality in MCOs?

16. What things do agencies such as NCQA and JCAHO typically look at in the accrediting process?

17. What is HEDIS?

18. What are TQM/CQI principles and why didn't they work well in managed care?

19. What is evidence-based medicine and what is the best "hierarchy of study design"?

20. What percent of medical problems are estimated to relate to lifestyle rather than genetic, environmental, or external factors?

21. Identify and describe three important tools that MCOs use to assess their members' health risks.

22. Why are employers often interested in the results of their employees' HRAs?

23. Identify and describe three intervention strategies MCOs might offer.

24. Why are Wellness Programs useful in managed care?

25. What are two alternative structures for Wellness Programs?

26. What factors must be examined and compared in reporting managed care results?

27. Name four reasons disease management is a logical approach to improving quality of care.

28. How do MCOs implement disease management programs?

29. Identify six elements of CIGNA HealthCare's diabetes disease management program.

30. What serves as an important source for an MCO to identify disease prevalence among its population?

31. What data do disease management programs specifically rely on?

32. Why might data be unavailable?

33. What five categories of care are subject to measurement by a disease management program?

34. What questions might a disease management program ask in analyzing its data and results?

35. What tools can MCOs use to protect the confidentiality of data, particularly in electronic transfer?

36. Why is reporting results in graphic form recommended?

37. How are disease management programs paid for?

38. Why are ethical and medicolegal issues relevant to disease management programs?

Chapter 15

MANAGING MARKET-DRIVEN ORGANIZATIONAL CHANGE

■ Key Terms

Business strategy

Buy-in

Change strategy

Comprehensive information systems

Core competencies

Cultural change

Eliminate redundancy

Leadership

Managing chronic care

Monitoring high cost/high risk

Multidisciplinary teams

Personal care plans

Population-based disease management

Reengineering process

Stakeholders

Treatment protocols

Use of new technology

Values

1. What effects are current market forces having on managed care?

2. Why do many people believe that tying financial incentives too closely to medical care creates ethical problems?

3. Identify four practices managed care's business values must adhere to for the system to remain effective.

4. Who are the "stakeholders" in managed care?

5. What six things must stakeholders do to create a partnership among managed care participants?

6. What are the most important resources an organization draws on in reengineering itself?

7. What individuals in managed care are most likely to challenge reengineering efforts?

8. Why is examining and defining corporate culture vital to successful reengineering?

9. Why is downsizing, which many people mistakenly consider reengineering, not a viable long-term business strategy?

10. What is reengineering and what is required for it to be successful?

11. What six questions must a health care organization resolve to successfully reorganize?

12. Why are these questions often viewed as a threat?

13. Give two examples of ways that reengineering forces health care organizations to change form and function.

14. What is the goal of management restructuring?

15. Why should individuals with direct contact with patients have more responsibility and authority?

16. How should services be evaluated for redundancy?

17. Who are most likely to become "system integrators"?

18. What is one key potential benefit of reengineering that is often ignored?

19. How can employers become involved in redesigning care delivery?

20. Where are core competencies vital?

21. How can technology help redesign health care?

22. Identify and describe the components necessary for the successful redesign of clinical systems and care delivery.

SAMPLE EXAMINATION

HIAA examinations may have three types of questions:

1) Positive Multiple Choice

Each question or statement below is followed by four answers lettered A, B, C, and D. Select the one answer which is best in each case. Completely fill in the bubble for the corresponding letters (A, B, C, or D) in the proper space on the answer sheet.

Sample Question:

The name of the ocean located between Europe and Africa on the east and North and South America on the west is the

   A. Arctic.
   B. Atlantic.*
   C. Indian.
   D. Pacific.

*Correct Answer.

2) Multiple Option

Each of the following questions contains an introduction followed by several expressions identified as I, II, and III. For each question, determine which one of the combinations identified as A, B, C, or D is most correct and completely fill in the bubble for the corresponding letter in the proper space on the answer sheet.

Sample Question:

Which of the states below border Canada?

   I. Alaska.
   II. Iowa.
   III. New York.

   A. III only
   B. I and II only
   C. I and III only*
   D. I, II, and III

*Correct Answer

Singular or plural grammatical form in the question does not imply a singular or plural answer. In the example, "Which of the states below border Canada?" the structure is plural, but the answer may be either singular (one state) or plural (two or more states).

3) Negative Multiple Choice

Each question is followed by four answers (A, B, C, and D). Select the answer which best completes the sentence and completely fill in the bubble for the corresponding letter (A, B, C, or D) in the proper space on the answer sheet.

Sample Question:

All the cities listed below are national capitals EXCEPT

    A. London.
    B. Paris.
    C. Sydney.*
    D. Washington.

*Correct Answer

The sample examination below (10 questions) is not meant to test your knowledge of the subject, but to show you the types of questions that might be asked. Do not use your score on this sample test to predict your score on the actual exam, since the number of questions is too few to be meaningful. The actual examination will contain 75 multiple choice questions, equally weighted, and have a time limit of two hours. HIAA examinations have been highly reliable in the past, almost always yielding reliability coefficients of .90 or better.

1. One of the advantages of collective employer arrangements with risk-bearing organizations is

    A. lower premium rates based on fewer employees.
    B. selective acceptance of an employer's insured individuals.
    C. rates typically guaranteed for three years based on more enrollees.
    D. more rigidity in the risk-bearer's approach to contract negotiations.

2. The DOD lacks military-owned or -operated facilities that are geographically accessible to every beneficiary. Therefore, the DOD

    A. relocates affected individuals.
    B. contracts with civilian providers on a regional basis.
    C. denies benefits to inaccessible individuals.
    D. transports affected individuals to military facilities for medical care.

3. Open-access plans differ from HMOs in that

    I. Patients can bypass gatekeepers to receive specialty care.
    II. Open-access plans impose a surcharge for self-referral.
    III. Patients can access any specialty provider they want.

    A. I and II only
    B. I, II, and III
    C. I and III only
    D. II and III only

4. The new Texas law, SB 386, provides that

    A. health carriers are immune from tort liability.
    B. health carriers are potentially subject to liability for damages caused by their employees' and agents' medical treatment decisions.

C. injured patients can only recover from a health carrier if they can prove the carrier intentionally caused the harm.

D. ERISA preempts all questions of state tort law.

5. Clara is a research scientist employed by the Food and Drug Administration. She would like to change her health care coverage from her current HMO to a more flexible POS plan. How can Clara change her coverage?

A. At any time by notifying the FDA payroll office.

B. Only during the Annual Open Season, which occurs each May-June.

C. She cannot change her coverage unless her employment status changes.

D. Only during Annual Open Season, which occurs every November-December.

6. What can MCOs do to improve, or in some cases maintain, their market position?

I. Become more competitive by raising premiums.

II. Create long-term strategic alliances with regional provider networks.

III. Reduce administrative expenses.

A. I, II, and III

B. I and III only

C. II and III only

D. II only

7. Recent polls show that the majority of Americans would prefer to see the health care industry regulated by

A. state governments.

B. insurance companies.

C. the federal government.

D. a nongovernmental entity.

8. TRICARE Prime most closely resembles

A. an HMO.

B. a PPO.

C. a POS.

D. a PSO.

9. MegaCare, Inc. is a large managed care organization operating in the Northeast. Dr. Jim Niceguy, a family physician with a small private practice in MidTown, has been trying unsuccessfully to become part of MegaCare's provider network. Assuming he meets MegaCare's participation requirements, Dr. Niceguy could require MegaCare to let him participate if his state has a(n)

A. mandatory point-of-service law.

B. any willing provider law.

C. anti-gag provision.

D. direct access law.

10. Typically, to be eligible to enroll in a Medicare+Choice plan, enrollees must

A. have reached the age of 55.

B. have reached the age of 65.

C. be entitled to Medicare Part A and enrolled in Part B.

D. be entitled to Medicare Part A but not enrolled in Part B.

■ Answers to Sample Test:

1. C
2. B
3. A
4. B
5. D
6. C
7. D
8. A
9. B
10. C